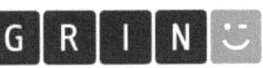

Bibliographic information published by the German National Library:

The German National Library lists this publication in the National Bibliography; detailed bibliographic data are available on the Internet at http://dnb.dnb.de .

Imprint:

Copyright © 2014 GRIN Verlag, Open Publishing GmbH
Print and binding: Books on Demand GmbH, Norderstedt Germany
ISBN: 978-3-668-15138-3

This book at GRIN:

http://www.grin.com/en/e-book/314821/diabetes-millitus-patients-within-minority-communities-cultural-and-lifestyle

Mercy Njiru

Diabetes Millitus Patients within Minority Communities. Cultural and Lifestyle Influences

GRIN Publishing

GRIN - Your knowledge has value

Since its foundation in 1998, GRIN has specialized in publishing academic texts by students, college teachers and other academics as e-book and printed book. The website www.grin.com is an ideal platform for presenting term papers, final papers, scientific essays, dissertations and specialist books.

Visit us on the internet:

http://www.grin.com/

http://www.facebook.com/grincom

http://www.twitter.com/grin_com

Developing Evidence based Practice:

Do Cultural and Local Lifestyle Influences Contribute in the Prevalence of New

Diagnosis Of DM?

Table of Contents

Abstract

The number of individuals belonging to minority communities is the US is increasing, and most of these communities are more susceptible to diabetes mellitus than other but majority populations. This could be because of genetic preference for diabetes mellitus and because of an unbalanced access to adequate healthcare. Therefore, understanding various cultural views is essential in providing healthcare for individuals in the minority communities within the US. The aim of this research is to find out the cultural and lifestyle influences on health of diabetes patients within minority communities. This paper achieves its objectives by examining 1) background research on the topic including statistics of diabetes mellitus among specific populations; 2) risk factors of diabetes mellitus amongst minority groups; 3) impact of cultural perceptions and lifestyle on diabetes mellitus care, and; 4) ways of reducing racial disparities in diabetes mellitus care. This proposed research ends with conclusions and recommendations on the topic.

Introduction

Diabetes mellitus (also referred to as Type Two diabetes) remains to be the seventh primary cause of deaths in the United States of America with a comparatively high mortality rate being found in the minority communities compared to the White majority. Some individuals, especially those belonging to some racial or ethnic minority communities can be at a certain risk in relation to getting effective diabetes mellitus care due to various reasons. Being a chronic illness, diabetes mellitus (DM) exhibits a disparate effect on individuals belonging to these racial or ethnic minority communities (Guthrie and Guthrie 2009). A higher preponderance for diabetes mellitus occurs among minority communities compared to the Whites. Consequently, some of these minority communities have very high rates of complications and deaths related to diabetes mellitus.

A national analysis conducted by the US Department of Health and Human Services provided important data showing that Mexican-American adults individuals were twice as likely as non-Hispanic white adults to get a diagnosis of diabetes mellitus by a doctor (Vinicor 2011). The Mexican-American minority community also had higher rates of older-stage nephritic disease related to diabetes mellitus as compared to their non-Hispanic white counterparts (Vinicor 2011). Apart from getting over the language and cultural barriers that are evident for minority groups, some of the diabetic patients may also be at risk of having culturally mistaken notion about healthcare givers in relation to diabetes mellitus. Additional research needs to be done among minority communities to determine if the strategies for promoting and supporting healthy lifestyles in relation to the management of diabetes mellitus are efficient.

Problem Statement

There have been relatively a few behavioral researches focusing on minority communities and diabetes mellitus. The accessibility to knowledge about diabetes mellitus among minority groups (such as African-Americans and Hispanics/Latinos) in the U.S has made it hard to curb the increasing prevalence and incidence of diabetes mellitus among these populations, and has hugely highlighted the significance of this issue in the public health. Previous and current researches have established that mutations within the insulin promoter factor–1 gene—the β-cell recording feature, which is crucial to pancreatic growth and sustenance of β-cell mass—increases vulnerability to type diabetes mellitus amongst the minority group of African-Americans (Poretsky 2010). On the contrary, the same genotype does not cause Type 2 diabetes or diabetes mellitus among White individuals.

Past investigations and findings indicate that Hispanics and Latinos are about 60% more likely to encounter deaths and complications related to diabetes mellitus compared to their non-Hispanic white counterparts (Talamantes, Lindeman, and Mouton n.d.). Diabetes mellitus is a rising epidemic among minority communities in America, especially the Hispanic or Latino and the African-America populations. There is an increase in the concern on increasing course of diabetes mellitus, especially among children and adolescents, specifically from the African-American and Hispanic communities, who are apparently at a greater risk of suffering from the disease.

Literature Review

Statistics

According to the statistics given by the National Institute of Diabetes and Digestive and Kidney Diseases (NIDDKD), an approximated 2.5 million American adults with Hispanic and Latino origins are diagnosed with diabetes mellitus. This is very overwhelming, considering that the number is about 9.5% of the entire Hispanic and Latino Americans' population. The report indicated that the minority community of Hispanic and Latino Americans are averagely 1.9 times more probable to get diabetes mellitus compared to non-Hispanic white individuals at the same age. In addition, the statistics indicated that an approximated 50% of children born of Hispanic and Latino family in 2000 were likely to get diabetes mellitus in the course of their lives (Franz, 2001).

The Center for Disease Control (CDC) data in 1995 indicated that minorities such as African- Americans, American-Indians, and Hispanics experienced a diabetes mortality rate of 19.3% to 28.5%, while the Caucasian-Americans rate was 11.7% (National Institutes of Health 2000). Notwithstanding the ages of individuals in a community or group, the overall health results for most minority Americans with diabetes mellitus seem to be suboptimal. Complications related to diabetes mellitus that face these minority communities include stroke and heart diseases, amputations, loss of sight, renal diseases, nervous system disease, and numerous life-threatening occurrences. These conditions remain grave worries for minority patients with diabetes mellitus. It has been noted that such grievous outcomes are experienced in these communities regardless of today's utilization rates and access to health care and screening of the complications of diabetes mellitus, hypertension, hyperglycemia, and dyslipidemia. The prevalence of diabetes mellitus amongst Hispanics is twice or thrice that of non-Hispanic Whites.

The occurrence of diabetes mellitus amongst various American-Indian groups varies from approximately 12% to more than 50%. The higher rate of this prevalence was documented in individuals aged 35 and above. According to a research report filed by the Strong Heart Study of American-Indians in four American states, prevalence rates of diabetes Mellitus was about 33% to 72%. After an adjustment in the age differences among the minority population, the 2007-2009 national survey statistics for individuals diagnosed with diabetes mellitus according to the prevalence by race and ethnicity include 11.8% being Hispanics; 12.6% of non-Hispanic blacks, 7.1% being non-Hispanic whites; and 8.4% of Asian-Americans (NDEP n.d.).

Risk Factors of Diabetes Mellitus amongst Minority Groups

A factor that has a great impact on the diabetes mellitus care for the minority populations in America is the absence of access to proper health care. This has greatly led to health disparities amongst these people. One of the major determining factors of access to quality healthcare is health insurance coverage. Other determinants include having basic healthcare facilities and having current contact with healthcare providers (Hurley 2010). The minority communities lack all these necessities completely, or have them but they are inadequate. Compared with individuals in other racial and ethnic groups, specifically the non-Hispanic whites, individuals from minority communities like the Hispanics and the American-Indians are more likely to lack healthcare insurance coverage. This is in accordance with the report published by the National Health Interview Survey conducted by the National Center for Health Statistics.

4

Additional research has found out that members from minority communities who suffer from diabetes mellitus are also faced by other economic barriers, which hinder their treatment. Research indicates that the economic status of the minority population in the United States is comparatively lower compared to the non-Hispanic white counterparts. This economic shortcoming has significant consequences on the health and healthcare of these minority populations. Particularly, in addition to being low-income earners, the Americans belonging to most minority groups, such as Hispanics or African-Americans, do not have health insurance coverage (Hurley 2010; Kahn and Joslin, 2005).

Impact of Cultural Perceptions and Lifestyle on Diabetes Mellitus Care

The minority population in the US is a combination of various communities including African-Americans, Latinos, and Hispanics. Hispanics include all individuals from Spanish-speaking nations, factoring in their cultural beliefs, their education, their values, and their socioeconomic status, while Latinos include all individuals from the Latin-American nations, which have different cultural beliefs, traditions, and values (Hurley 2010). These minority communities are a composition of many different cultures and some minor similarities amongst them. For instance, for the Hispanics and the Latinos' culture, family is imperative and can affect an individual's healthcare practices. Research demonstrates that family significant support accorded by family is vital in warranting patient's adherence to diabetes mellitus management activities. The lack of family support gives patients less motivation to manage diabetes mellitus properly. Managing an intricate chronic disease such as diabetes touches on the suffering individual and his or her family members since it involves much knowledge and responsibilities, and sometimes painful complications, such as amputations, blindness, and heart diseases.

Some of the minority communities have a laid-back perspective on life and some actually consider diabetes mellitus to be the result of divine mediation; while others use traditional medicine to treat diabetes mellitus. In an analysis of 104 adult patients from the Hispanic community, 78% of them claimed diabetes mellitus was due to God's will, while 17% used herbaceous plants to cure the condition. Thus, experts suggest that it is imperative to understand the religious and spiritual perceptions of patients when addressing the issue of diabetes mellitus and other health issues in the minority population.

Reducing Racial Disparities in Diabetes Mellitus Care

Getting rid of the cultural disparity from diabetes mellitus patients in different communities strongly relies upon various things, including effective communication with patients in a preferred, culturally competent way and increasing the patients' literacy about health. A research program funded by Agency for Healthcare Research and Quality (AHRQ) established ways through which racial and ethnic prevalence of diabetes mellitus can be cut down (Narayan 2011). Approaches of preventing the inception of diabetes mellitus through changing lifestyles involve interventions, which may be ethnically sensitive and specific to populations, but can also be helpful. Clinicians should be culturally competent and capable of changing their individual beliefs and attitudes and focus on the patient in order to achieve the best medical results, irrespective of the background of the patient. The physician must establish a connection with patients, bearing in mind the perspective of patients on disease management and medication.

Healthcare providers should enhance effectiveness in communication since diabetes mellitus is a complex condition calling for changes in the lifestyle of patients. Accordingly, patients have to be plainly informed of the different aspects of managing diabetes mellitus. Patients should be made to understand the importance of proper diet, continuous monitoring, and exercise. This ought to be achieved through all possible means, including the use of family member interpreters or other interpreters to communicate this information to the patients. Healthcare centers should also employ staff members who are multilingual in order to help patients feel comfortable during their office visits. Diabetes mellitus advocates should also be involved in such activities as educating the patients, offering outreach programs, screening populations, and managing diabetes mellitus cases (Daugirdas and Blake 2007).

Understanding and decreasing healthcare discrepancies can assist develop better health results for diabetes mellitus patients belonging to minority groups. Effectiveness in communication by healthcare providers and other efforts of improving health knowledge amongst diabetes mellitus patients can bring about improvements in management of the disease. Consequently, this can place an emphasis on realizing glycemic regulation and decreasing the risk for complications related to diabetes mellitus. A good understanding of ethnic variances and the influence on healthcare greatly affect the services provided by clinicians to diabetic patients belonging to minority community. Consequently, this would lead to results that help lessen the ethnic divide in diabetes mellitus care.

Research Question

The key focus of this study will be to answer the question: Does cultural and local lifestyle influences contribute in the prevalence of new diagnosis of diabetes mellitus?

Methodology

To answer the study question, the researcher will utilize an appropriate, academically proven methodology. The researcher will use a qualitative research design to explore to find out whether cultural and local lifestyle influences contribute in the prevalence of new diagnosis of diabetes mellitus. The research will compare incidences, complications, and deaths between clients from the minority groups (Blacks, Asian Americans, American Indians, Hawaiians, and Hispanics) and whites. Qualitative study is a system of inquiry that attempts to build a general, largely narrative, account to communicate the researcher's realizing of a social or cultural phenomenon. A qualitative approach of study takes place in natural circumstances utilizing a blend of reflections, interviews, and document analyses. This study approach is largely an inductive practice of categorizing data and distinguishing patterns or relationships among the categories.

The researcher will primarily base this study on previous studies, reports, and case studies, while bearing in mind that in a case study, a single organization, program, phenomenon, process, institution, or event is looked into within a determined period, using a blend of suitable data collection methods. In this study, the research will separately dig into the information regarding minority groups (Blacks, Asian Americans, American Indians, Hawaiians, and Hispanics) and whites concerning diabetes mellitus. A case study design will be applicable to this research, since habitually, case studies are used in medicine, law, and most importantly in healthcare studies. However, for a case study methodology to be effective, it requires most of these five components: Study questions, assumptions (if any); unit of analysis, the logic connecting data to the assumptions, and; the criteria for interpretation of the findings. The researcher will ensure the application of at least four of these five elements.

A case study research design may result in a more informal ground for theory development through analytical rather than pure statistical inductions. Besides, a theory can give a perceptual experience and a manner of considering an interpretation, which eventually brings about the understanding of some phenomenon. For that reason, the researcher will prefer a case study to better explore, if any, the differences in incidences, complications, and deaths among the US minority groups and whites. There are some approaches of relating data to assumptions, and one of them is pattern matching, which the researcher intends to use for this proposed study.

Following the pattern-matching approach before the actual research, the researcher will develop opposing propositions, before developing several pieces of information from the exploration, in relation to the opposing theoretical propositions. In addition, the researcher will incorporate the following elements in the qualitative research design to establish whether cultural and local lifestyle influences contribute to the prevalence of new diagnosis of diabetes mellitus—research questions; scope of study; unit of analysis; selection of a case; data collection; method of analysis, and; tests for design quality.

Study Population

The researcher will comprise individuals who will be asked to willingly sign up at the beginning of the study. They will be signed up individually at 15 healthcare facilities set up by the government to offer healthcare services to individuals living within low-income areas and in selected hospitals in different areas across the states of Arizona, Florida, Chicago, Louisiana, Maine, and Vermont. Participants from African-American, Hispanic, and Latino ethnic groups will be registered at the community health centers within their states, while the White participants will be enrolled in the selected hospitals within the states. The enrollment of the participants will be conducted in a random approach. The participants who will be eligible for the study are expected to be between the ages of 34 and 80 years, and interested in participating in the study.

Data Collection

Still in answering the main research question, the researcher will use the semi-structured interviews data collection method, to obtain information that will supplement cases studies. The semi-structured interview method is widely the most common form of interviewing, probably why the researcher knows about it. The method will involve the researcher working as an interviewer following a set of already prepared set of questions. However, the interview will be made colloquial/conversational. This method will enable the researcher to change the order of the pre-written questions or the way the questions are written as the interview goes on, to keep the questions relevant and interview organized. With the semi-structured interview, the researcher can give explanations or omit questions that may seem pleonastic or redundant. Therefore, the researcher will be able to make the interviewee talk at will and responsively, providing in-depth information.

To use the semi-structured interview to collect data successively, the researcher intends to:

i.   Listen carefully to the interviewee; ensure that questions are short, direct and clear;

ii.   Remain neutral through the interview; enjoy the interview to make the interviewee comfortable in answering questions;

iii.   Use probes and prompts to obtain as much information as possible, and;

iv.   Take an entire record of the interview, either by audio recording or by transcription.

During the days of the interviews, the researcher will follow the following steps:

i.   Introduce oneself as a researcher;

ii.   Warm up the interviewee by asking some easy, friendly questions at the beginning to make the interviewee feel comfortable;

iii.   Perform the interview logically; 'cool off', i.e. Ask a few straightforward questions at the end the interview to calm the interviewee, and;

iv.   Eventually show gratitude and bid the interviewees goodbye.

The researcher will use the semi-structured interview method because it is less pushy to interviewees, not to mention it promotes two-way communication (between the interviewer and the interviewee). Interviewees can freely ask questions of the researcher (interviewer), which makes the semi-structured interview method work as an extension tool as well. Participants will be required to undergo a comprehensive, personal interview that will touch of different facets of health and conduct such as individual and family medical history, nutrition, workouts, use of medicine, societal support, and health services access. During the interview, participants will encounter some closed questions, such as, "did you personally decide to test for diabetes or high blood sugar?" and according to their responses, 'yes or no', the participants will be asked follow-up questions on subjects such as what age they were diagnosed and what, and how they use prescription medications to manage their diabetes.

Ethical Considerations

Various ethical issues will be considered for this study, including discretion of information, informant safety, and informed consent. The informants will be provided with information sheets that explain the purpose of the study ahead of involving them in interviews. The researcher will also enlighten the informants of what they will need to participate in the study as interviewees. In addition, the informants in the interview will be given time to willingly decide if they will participate in the interview. Individual participation in this study will be based on voluntary and by informed consent. According to Miller and Bell (2002), it is a requirement rather than a trusting verbal consent that researchers obtain written consent from the people, particularly informants, whom they involve in their studies.

The issues of confidentiality for this study will be dealt with as part of the process of informed consent. Details on the manner in which data confidentiality will be kept will be printed on the information sheet that will be provided to the informants, which according to Oliver (2003), will be expected to help to keep up with best practice rules. Data that will be collected for this study will be treated while keeping in mind the requirements of confidentiality. The digital data that will be used to store the digital recorder and the computer will be protected by use of a password, while the data in paper records will be kept in locked filing cabinets. Another measure will be that only the researcher will be responsible for handling both forms of data, and hence the only one that will be having access to these data even after the study. Once the study will be concluded, the researcher will keep the audio recordings and notes while ensuring these media will not reveal identities of the informants giving some sensitive information.

The anonymity of the informants will be safeguarded and no individual will be identified by name or otherwise at any one point during the study, especially on written reports. Accordingly, the transcripts from the interview will each allocated a code. This code will be used in referring to the transcript when presenting their quotations in the report of findings. However, the researcher is aware the use of codes for names will not an easy task, and ensuring anonymity of the participants will even be more difficult. In that regard, the researcher will take extra care to avoid revealing personal information concerning the informants, or using quotations that would make the informants recognizable in any way. In cases where the researcher will use names, job title, or affiliations, the identities will not be actual for the reasons given hereabout.

Proposed Data Analysis Method and Presentation

The researcher recognizes the fact that most methodologies of qualitative data analysis tend to share partly the same analytic processes. These processes involve what the researcher will follow for this study:

10

i.   After collecting data, the first step of analysis will be going through it (the data);

ii.   Then reading the data and annotating it, and finally;

iii.   Identifying specific items of interest.

These three steps are typically known as coding, and by them, the first major analytic phase for the researcher will involve coding the data—or simply, following through the three steps. Through the coding process, the researcher will define what the collected data are about. The coded data from semi-structured interviews will be compared with the information obtained from cases studies and relevant literature review to show any similarities or differences from earlier studies. To present the collected and analyzed data, the researcher will use tables and graphs. However, the two most significant means will be quotations and statements from the semi-structured interviews. Wherever the researcher will directly quote the source or interviewee, the "" marks will be used.

Expected Results

According to the research that the has already been done, the researcher expects the majority of the participants from the minority communities to report a comparatively low household income, and comparatively low number of schooling years. The researcher also anticipates that amongst most of the diabetes mellitus patients, most of them will be overweight, or have an extreme prevalence for obese. Across all the communities, the researcher anticipates that the most of the sufferers to be women than men. Generally, the research anticipates that to observe the prejudiced socioeconomic and other disadvantageous factors are a huge contribution towards the prevalence of diabetes mellitus amongst the minorities.

Discussion of Findings in Relation To Literature

After analyzing and presenting data, the researcher will be interested in knowing if this study's findings are the same or different from other researchers', especially those published in the examined case studies. Accordingly, the research will compare this study's findings with the available literature that explores the differences and similarities of the incidences, complications, and deaths between and among the minority groups and whites. This step will also contribute in validating this research's findings. The researcher will also emphasize the unique findings, if any, from other existing pieces of literature. Another aspect the research will be discussing is whether there are factors, such as time, which would have affected the findings.

Limitations

There may be occurrences of systematic erroneousness in reporting diabetes mellitus diagnoses, thus obscuring actual racial disparities in the study. However, data collection in a consistent manner should reduce this possibility. Non-differential misclassification can also reduce real differences in the reported results but substantially produce a null finding. The research will be based on the prevalence of diabetes mellitus on the minorities and not necessarily on the issue of undiagnosed incidences of the. Thus, reasons why we may experience null findings as self-reports on this issue have been used in previous studies to document strong racial/ethnic discrepancies.

Conclusion and Recommendations

Within the United States, diabetes mellitus issue is of importance to the public health for all racial/ethnic groups. Nonetheless, there is call for addressing this issue especially within the minority populations. The prevalence of diabetes mellitus is hard to define since different measures are used and generally, experts consider 1% to 2% prevalence within the general population reasonable. Some researchers report that in particular ethnic groups the disease prevalence could reach 50%, with some of the highest prevalence being found amongst Mexican-Americans and Non-Hispanic Blacks. The current research concentrating on diabetes mellitus amongst minority communities has brought about new understandings regarding the variability in medical indexes. New intervention approaches formulated to decrease the prevalent levels of complications related to diabetes mellitus among minorities have to consider the psychosocial and the socioeconomic factors contributing to poor follow of diabetes mellitus management approaches.

Data on the epidemiology and effects of diabetes mellitus amongst minority communities propose numerous key requirements, including identifying features liable for the increasing occurrence of noninsulin-dependent diabetes mellitus (NIDDM) in minority populations. These include determining the etiology of the uncommon type of diabetes mellitus amongst minority communities; handling the high morbidity and mortality rates related to the prevalence of diabetes mellitus amongst minority communities; and defining the explanations for the high prevalence of risk factors that are associated with diabetes amongst minority communities, especially hypertension and obesity (Thomas, Nelson, and Silverman 2005).

12

Bibliography

Daugirdas, J. T., Blake, P. G., & Ing, T. S. (2007). *Handbook of dialysis* (4th ed.). Philadelphia: Lippincott Williams & Wilkins.

Diabetes and Pre-diabetes Statistics and Facts | NDEP. (n.d.). *National Diabetes Education Program - Free Information to Prevent and Control Diabetes | NDEP.* Retrieved October 18, 2011, from http://ndep.nih.gov/diabetes-facts/index.aspx

Franz, M. (2001). Medical Nutrition Therapy for Diabetes Mellitus and Hypoglycemia of Nondiabetic Origin. *Medical Nutrition Therapy.*

Guthrie, D. W., & Guthrie, R. A. (2009). *Management of diabetes mellitus: a guide to the pattern approach /* (6th ed.). New York: Springer Pub. Co..

Hurley, D. (2010). *Diabetes rising: how a rare disease became a modern pandemic, and what to do about it.* Bangkok: Kaplan Pub..

Kahn, C. R., & Joslin, E. P. (2005). *Joslin's diabetes mellitus* (14th ed.). Philadelphia: Lippincott Williams & Willkins.

Miller, T. and Bell, L. (2002). Consenting to what? Issues of access, gate-keeping and 'informed' consent. In Mauthner, M., Birch, M., Jessop, J. & Miller, T. *Ethics in Qualitative Research* London: Sage.

Narayan, K. M. (2011). *Diabetes public health: from data to policy.* London: Oxford University Press.

National Institutes of Health. (2000, June 27). NIH Guide: Diabetes Self-Management in Minority Populations. *OER Home Page - Grants Web Site.* Retrieved October 18, 2011, from http://grants.nih.gov/grants/guide/pa-files/PA-00-113.html

Oliver P (2003). *The Student's Guide to Research Ethics*, Maidenhead and Philadelphia, PA: Open University Press.

Poretsky, L. (2010). *Principles of Diabetes Mellitus* (2nd ed.). Berlin and Heidelberg: Springer Verlag.

Talamantes, M., Lindeman, R., & Mouton, C. (n.d.). Health and Health care of Hispanic/Latino American. *Stanford University.* Retrieved October 18, 2011, from http://www.stanford.edu/group/ethnoger/hispaniclatino.html

Thomas, J. R., Nelson, J. K., & Silverman, S. J. (2005). *Research methods in physical activity* (5th ed.). Champaign, IL: Human Kinetics.

Vinicor, F. (n.d.). CDC - Diabetes and Women's Health Across the Life Stages - Publications - Diabetes DDT. *Centers for Disease Control and Prevention.*

Retrieved October 18, 2011, from

http://www.cdc.gov/diabetes/pubs/women/index.htm

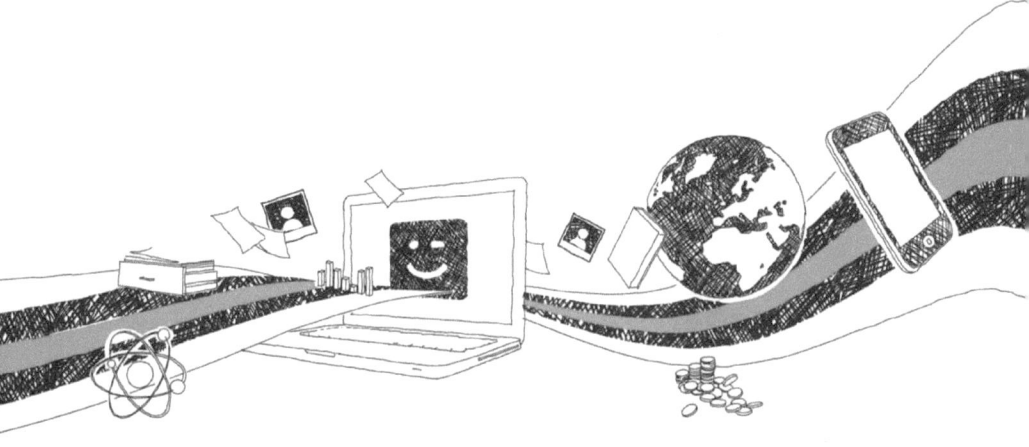
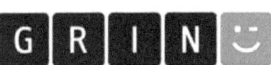